ANTHONOGY

OF

AWESOMENESS

Created by Duncan Sailors

CONTENTS

Our Vision

Strengthen our Community.

The Mission

Build a fitness driven community in downtown Seattle for anyone looking to move, look, feel, and live better through professionally guided training.

Our Core Values

1. Community Driven
2. Daily success
3. Continual learning

How to Use the Weekly Log

1. Write the day in the **DAY** box.

2. Write the date in the **DATE** box.

3. In the area below the day and date, write the workout(s) that you do for that day. Make sure to include all information about the workout; exercises, sets, reps, load, rounds, scaling, time….any information that will allow you to repeat the same workout at a later time. Also, write any notes regarding how the workout felt, problems with movements (the ques your trainer keeps yelling at you), PR's, actions that you take for recovery, etc.

4. In the **NOTES** box, write any data or notes that do not apply to a given day.

EXAMPLE:

<table>
<tr><td colspan="2">MONDAY   12/12/14</td></tr>
<tr><td colspan="2">foam roller, dynamic stretching</td></tr>
<tr><td>Back Squat 5 x 5</td><td>5 rounds of:</td></tr>
<tr><td>5 @ 40 kg</td><td>200m row</td></tr>
<tr><td>5 @ 44kg</td><td>7 DB push press @ #15</td></tr>
<tr><td>5 @ 50 kg</td><td>7 KB deadlift @ 24kg</td></tr>
<tr><td>5 @ 55 kg</td><td>7 knees to chest</td></tr>
<tr><td>3 @ 60 kg - hard!</td><td>18:27 - tired and</td></tr>
<tr><td>brace! knees out!</td><td>sore!</td></tr>
</table>

How to Use the Benchmark Workout Log

In the Benchmark Workout Log section you can keep track of workouts and training events that you repeat frequently (ie. 2000m row), or any workout with a name (ie. Helen).

Make sure to record how you scaled the workout and any notes about the workout.

EXAMPLE:

Helen	Rx	Load/Scale	Time/Rounds	Load/Scale	Time/Rounds
3 rounds of:			7/15/12		11/15/12
400m run					
21 kb swings	24kg	16 kg	13:42	16kg	12:53
12 pullups		purple band		black band	PR!

LEVEL 1   well rounded beginner

Created by Dave Werner

Qualified/Date

hips	air squats	100 reps	
push	pushups	20 reps	
pull	static hang	30 seconds	
core	sit ups	30 reps	
work	kettlebell swings	25 reps	
speed	400m run	2:04 minutes	
hips	deadlift	3/4 x bodyweight	
push	military press	1/4 x bodyweight	
pull	medicine ball cleans	10 reps	
core	knees to chest	10 reps sitting	
work	wall ball	25 reps	
work	800m run	4:20 minutes	
speed	500m row	m 1:55, w 2:20	
hips	vertical jump	10 inches	
push	dips	3 reps	
pull	pull ups	3 reps	
core	L-sit	10 seconds	
work	2000m row	m 8:10, w 9:50	
speed	dumbbell snatch	10/arm	
work	Christine	15 minutes	
work	1 mile run	9 minutes	
skill	barbell clean	demonstrate technique	
skill	barbell snatch	demonstrate technique	
skill	front squat	demonstrate technique	
skill	overhead squat	demonstrate technique	
skill	thruster	demonstrate technique	
skill	KB clean/snatch	demonstrate technique	
pull	kipping pull up	demonstrate technique	
work	burpee	demonstrate technique	

Level 1 Qualified

LEVEL 2   intermediate athlete

Created by Dave Werner

Qualified/Date

hips	air squats	100 reps	__________________
hips	back squat	1 x bodyweight	__________________
push	pushups	30 reps	__________________
push	bench press	1 x bodyweight	__________________
pull	rope climb	20 feet, 1 trip	__________________
core	v-up	30 reps	__________________
work	kettlebell snatch	30/arm m24kg, w16kg	__________________
speed	400m run	1:34 minutes	__________________
hips	deadlift	1 1/2 x bodyweight	__________________
push	military press	1/4 x bodyweight	__________________
push	handstand hold	1 minute	__________________
pull	power clean	3/4 x bodyweight	__________________
core	hanging K2E	15 reps	__________________
work	thruster	45 reps @ 1/2 bodyweight	__________________
work	800m run	3:20 minutes	__________________
speed	500m row	m1:45, w2:00	__________________
hips	vertical jump	18 inches	__________________
push	dips	20 reps	__________________
push	dips	1 @ 1/3 bodyweight	__________________
pull	pull ups	20 reps	__________________
pull	pull ups	1 @ 1/3 bodyweight	__________________
pull	muscle up	1 rep	__________________
core	L-sit	30 seconds	__________________
work	2000m row	m7:30, w8:50	__________________
speed	power snatch	1/2 bodyweight	__________________
work	Helen	11:30 minutes	__________________
work	1 mile run	7 minutes	__________________

Level 2 Qualified __________________

LEVEL 3　　advanced athlete

Created by Dave Werner

			Qualified/Date
hips	pistols	10/leg	_______________
hips	back squat	1 1/2 x bodyweight	_______________
push	pushups	40 on rings	_______________
push	bench press	1 1/4 x bodyweight	_______________
pull	rope climb	20 feet, 1 trip, no feet	_______________
core	overhead squat	1 x bodyweight	_______________
work	kettlebell snatch	10 minute test, 200 reps m24kg, w16kg	_______________
speed	400m run	1:19 minutes	_______________
hips	deadlift	2 x bodyweight	_______________
push	military press	3/4 x bodyweight	_______________
push	handstand push up	10 reps	_______________
pull	clean	1 x bodyweight	_______________
core	hanging straight leg raise	20 reps	_______________
work	sandbag carry	1 mile, 1/2 x bodyweight	_______________
work	800m run	2:50 minutes	_______________
speed	500m row	m1:32, w1:50	_______________
hips	vertical jump	25 inches	_______________
push	dips	30 reps on rings	_______________
push	dips	1 @ 3/4 bodyweight	_______________
pull	pull ups	40 reps	_______________
pull	pull ups	1 @ 3/4 bodyweight	_______________
pull	muscle up	10 reps	_______________
core	L-sit	1 minute	_______________
work	5k row for women	21 minutes	_______________
work	6k row for men	21:45 minutes	_______________
speed	snatch	1 x bodyweight	_______________
work	Chelsea	All rounds completed	_______________
work	1 mile run	6 minutes	_______________

Level 3 Qualified　__________________________

Created by Dave Werner

hips	pistols	25/leg	_________________
hips	back squat	2 x bodyweight	_________________
push	pushups	60 on rings	_________________
push	bench press	1 1/2 x bodyweight	_________________
pull	rope climb	20 feet, 2 trips, no feet	_________________
core	overhead squat	15 reps @ bodyweight	_________________
work	2 db clean & jerk	10 min, 150 reps	
		m24kg, w16kg	_________________
speed	400m run	1:04 minutes	_________________
hips	deadlift	2 1/2 x bodyweight	_________________
push	military press	1 x bodyweight	_________________
push	handstand push up	10 reps	_________________
pull	clean	1 1/2 x bodyweight	_________________
core	front lever	15 seconds	_________________
work	sandbag carry	1 mile, 3/4 x bodyweight	_________________
work	800m run	2:20 minutes	_________________
speed	500m row	m1:25, w1:40	_________________
hips	vertical jump	30 inches	_________________
push	dips	50 reps on rings	_________________
push	dips	1 @ 1 x bodyweight	_________________
pull	pull ups	40 deadhang	_________________
pull	pull ups	1 @ 1 x bodyweight	_________________
pull	muscle up	15 reps	_________________
core	L-sit	1:30 minute	_________________
work	5k row for women	20 minutes	_________________
work	6k row for men	20 minutes	_________________
speed	snatch	1 1/4 x bodyweight	_________________
work	Mary	15 Rounds	_________________
work	1 mile run	5 minutes	_________________

Level 4 Qualified   _________________

DAY   DATE

DAY   DATE

DAY
DATE

DAY
DATE

DAY ___________ DATE __________

DAY ___________ DATE __________

DAY
DATE
DAY
DATE

DAY
DATE

DAY
DATE

DAY | DATE

DAY | DATE

DAY
DATE

DAY
DATE

DAY   DATE

DAY   DATE

DAY   DATE

DAY   DATE

DAY   DATE

DAY   DATE

DAY DATE

DAY DATE

DAY   DATE

DAY   DATE

DAY DATE

DAY DATE

DAY   DATE

DAY   DATE

DAY   DATE

DAY   DATE

DAY
DATE

DAY
DATE

DAY DATE

DAY DATE

DAY   DATE

DAY   DATE

DAY   DATE

DAY   DATE

DAY   DATE

DAY   DATE

DAY   DATE

DAY   DATE

DAY   DATE

DAY   DATE

DAY   DATE

DAY   DATE

DAY
DATE
DAY
DATE

DAY   DATE

DAY   DATE

DAY   DATE

DAY   DATE

DAY

DATE

DAY

DATE

DAY   DATE

DAY   DATE

DAY
DATE
DAY
DATE

DAY   DATE

DAY   DATE

DAY   DATE

DAY   DATE

DAY   DATE

DAY   DATE

DAY DATE

DAY DATE

DAY   DATE

DAY   DATE

DAY   DATE

DAY   DATE

DAY   DATE

DAY   DATE

DAY   DATE

DAY   DATE

DAY   DATE

DAY   DATE

DAY DATE

DAY DATE

DAY   DATE

DAY   DATE

DAY

DATE

DAY

DATE

DAY DATE

DAY DATE

DAY   DATE

DAY   DATE

DAY
DATE

DAY
DATE

DAY DATE

DAY DATE

DAY   DATE

DAY   DATE

DAY   DATE

DAY   DATE

DAY   DATE

DAY   DATE

DAY   DATE

DAY   DATE

DAY   DATE

DAY   DATE

DAY ______ DATE ______

DAY ______ DATE ______

DAY   DATE

DAY   DATE

DAY   DATE

DAY   DATE

DAY   DATE

DAY   DATE

DAY	DATE

DAY	DATE

DAY DATE

DAY DATE

DAY   DATE

DAY   DATE

DAY   DATE

DAY   DATE

DAY DATE

DAY DATE

DAY   DATE

DAY   DATE

DAY   DATE

DAY   DATE

DAY
DATE

DAY
DATE

DAY
DATE

DAY
DATE

DAY   DATE

DAY   DATE

DAY   DATE

DAY   DATE

DAY   DATE

DAY   DATE

DAY   DATE

DAY   DATE

DAY   DATE

DAY   DATE

DAY
DATE

DAY
DATE

DAY   DATE

DAY   DATE

DAY   DATE

DAY   DATE

DAY   DATE

DAY   DATE

DAY
DATE
DAY
DATE

DAY   DATE

DAY   DATE

DAY | DATE

DAY | DATE

DAY ___________ DATE

DAY ___________ DATE

DAY   DATE

DAY   DATE

DAY   DATE

DAY   DATE

DAY   DATE

DAY   DATE

DAY   DATE

DAY   DATE

BENCHMARK LOG

NAME	Rx	Load/Scale	Time/Rounds	Load/Scale	Time/Rounds
			DATE		DATE
NAME	Rx	Load/Scale	Time/Rounds	Load/Scale	Time/Rounds
			DATE		DATE
NAME	Rx	Load/Scale	Time/Rounds	Load/Scale	Time/Rounds
			DATE		DATE
NAME	Rx	Load/Scale	Time/Rounds	Load/Scale	Time/Rounds
			DATE		DATE
NAME	Rx	Load/Scale	Time/Rounds	Load/Scale	Time/Rounds
			DATE		DATE

Load/Scale	Time/Rounds	Load/Scale	Time/Rounds	Notes
	DATE		DATE	
Load/Scale	Time/Rounds	Load/Scale	Time/Rounds	Notes
	DATE		DATE	
Load/Scale	Time/Rounds	Load/Scale	Time/Rounds	Notes
	DATE		DATE	
Load/Scale	Time/Rounds	Load/Scale	Time/Rounds	Notes
	DATE		DATE	
Load/Scale	Time/Rounds	Load/Scale	Time/Rounds	Notes
	DATE		DATE	

BENCHMARK LOG

NAME	Rx	Load/Scale	Time/Rounds	Load/Scale	Time/Rounds
NAME			DATE		DATE
NAME	Rx	Load/Scale	Time/Rounds	Load/Scale	Time/Rounds
NAME			DATE		DATE
NAME	Rx	Load/Scale	Time/Rounds	Load/Scale	Time/Rounds
NAME			DATE		DATE
NAME	Rx	Load/Scale	Time/Rounds	Load/Scale	Time/Rounds
NAME			DATE		DATE
NAME	Rx	Load/Scale	Time/Rounds	Load/Scale	Time/Rounds
NAME			DATE		DATE

Load/Scale	Time/Rounds	Load/Scale	Time/Rounds	Notes
	DATE		DATE	
	DATE		DATE	
	DATE		DATE	
	DATE		DATE	
	DATE		DATE	

BENCHMARK LOG

NAME	Rx	Load/Scale	Time/Rounds	Load/Scale	Time/Rounds
			DATE		DATE
NAME	Rx	Load/Scale	Time/Rounds	Load/Scale	Time/Rounds
			DATE		DATE
NAME	Rx	Load/Scale	Time/Rounds	Load/Scale	Time/Rounds
			DATE		DATE
NAME	Rx	Load/Scale	Time/Rounds	Load/Scale	Time/Rounds
			DATE		DATE
NAME	Rx	Load/Scale	Time/Rounds	Load/Scale	Time/Rounds
			DATE		DATE

BENCHMARK LOG

Load/Scale	Time/Rounds	Load/Scale	Time/Rounds	Notes
	DATE		DATE	
	DATE		DATE	
	DATE		DATE	
	DATE		DATE	
	DATE		DATE	

BENCHMARK LOG

NAME	Rx	Load/Scale	Time/Rounds	Load/Scale	Time/Rounds
			DATE		DATE
NAME	Rx	Load/Scale	Time/Rounds	Load/Scale	Time/Rounds
			DATE		DATE
NAME	Rx	Load/Scale	Time/Rounds	Load/Scale	Time/Rounds
			DATE		DATE
NAME	Rx	Load/Scale	Time/Rounds	Load/Scale	Time/Rounds
			DATE		DATE
NAME	Rx	Load/Scale	Time/Rounds	Load/Scale	Time/Rounds
			DATE		DATE

Load/Scale	Time/Rounds	Load/Scale	Time/Rounds	Notes
	DATE		DATE	
Load/Scale	Time/Rounds	Load/Scale	Time/Rounds	Notes
	DATE		DATE	
Load/Scale	Time/Rounds	Load/Scale	Time/Rounds	Notes
	DATE		DATE	
Load/Scale	Time/Rounds	Load/Scale	Time/Rounds	Notes
	DATE		DATE	
Load/Scale	Time/Rounds	Load/Scale	Time/Rounds	Notes
	DATE		DATE	

DOUBLE UNDERS

1 minute		2 minutes		5 minutes		10 minutes	
DATE	REPS	DATE	REPS	DATE	REPS	DATE	REPS

AWESOME CYCLE

1 minute		3 minutes		5 minutes		10 minutes	
DATE	REPS	DATE	REPS	DATE	REPS	DATE	REPS

500m ROW

DATE	TIME

DATE	TIME

DATE	TIME

1000m ROW

DATE	TIME

DATE	TIME

2000m ROW

DATE	TIME

DATE	TIME

5000m ROW

DATE	SPLIT	TIME

10000m ROW

DATE	SPLIT	TIME

DATE	REPS	LOAD		DATE	REPS	LOAD		DATE	REPS	LOAD

THRUSTER

DATE	REPS	LOAD		DATE	REPS	LOAD		DATE	REPS	LOAD

CLEAN

DATE	REPS	LOAD		DATE	REPS	LOAD		DATE	REPS	LOAD

POWER CLEAN

DATE	REPS	LOAD		DATE	REPS	LOAD		DATE	REPS	LOAD

SNATCH

DATE	REPS	LOAD		DATE	REPS	LOAD		DATE	REPS	LOAD

POWER SNATCH

DATE	REPS	LOAD		DATE	REPS	LOAD		DATE	REPS	LOAD

BENCH PRESS

DATE	REPS	LOAD	DATE	REPS	LOAD	DATE	REPS	LOAD

CLOSE GRIP BENCH PRESS

DATE	REPS	LOAD	DATE	REPS	LOAD	DATE	REPS	LOAD

PUSH JERK

DATE	REPS	LOAD	DATE	REPS	LOAD	DATE	REPS	LOAD

SPLIT JERK

DATE	REPS	LOAD	DATE	REPS	LOAD	DATE	REPS	LOAD

PRESS

DATE	REPS	LOAD	DATE	REPS	LOAD	DATE	REPS	LOAD

PUSH PRESS

DATE	REPS	LOAD	DATE	REPS	LOAD	DATE	REPS	LOAD

OVERHEAD SQUAT

DATE	REPS	LOAD	DATE	REPS	LOAD	DATE	REPS	LOAD

DEADLIFT

DATE	REPS	LOAD	DATE	REPS	LOAD	DATE	REPS	LOAD

BACK SQUAT

DATE	REPS	LOAD		DATE	REPS	LOAD		DATE	REPS	LOAD

FRONT SQUAT

DATE	REPS	LOAD		DATE	REPS	LOAD		DATE	REPS	LOAD

SKIN FOLD MEASUREMENTS

DATE	BODYWEIGHT	CHEEK	CHIN	PEC/HAMSTRING	TRICEPS	SUBSCAP	MIDAXILLA	SUPRAILIAC	UMBILIAC	THIGH	CALF	TOTAL SUM	MIDSECTION SUM		

SKIN FOLD MEASUREMENTS

DATE	BODYWEIGHT	CHEEK	CHIN	PEC/HAMSTRING	TRICEPS	SUBSCAP	MIDAXILLA	SUPRAILIAC	UMBILIAC	THIGH	CALF	TOTAL SUM	MIDSECTION SUM		

www.ingramcontent.com/pod-product-compliance
Lightning Source LLC
Chambersburg PA
CBHW050920260726
48660CB00001B/301